C000165588

The Ultimate Guide to Plant-Based Breakfast

A Complete Collection of Breakfast Recipes to Start Your Plant-Based Diet and Improve Your Health

Dave Ingram

Table of contents

Ultimate Breakfast Burrito

Prep time: 5 minutes

Cook time: 20 minutes

Serves 2

Ingredients:

½ block (7 ounces / 198 g) firm tofu

2 medium potatoes, cut into ¼-inch dice

1 cup cooked black beans 4 ounces (113 g) mushrooms, sliced

1 jalapeño, seeded and diced

2 tablespoons vegetable broth or water 1 tablespoon nutritional yeast

½ teaspoon garlic powder

½ teaspoon onion powder

¼ cup salsa

6 corn tortillas

Directions:

1.   Heat a large skillet over medium-low heat.

2.   Drain the tofu, then place it in the pan and mash it down with a fork or mixing spoon.

3.   Stir the potatoes, black beans, mushrooms, jalapeño, broth, nutritional yeast, garlic powder, and onion powder into the skillet. Let it cook for 10 minutes, or until the potatoes can be easily pierced with a fork.

4.   Uncover and stir in the salsa. Stir well.

5.   Warm the tortillas until soft.

6.   Remove the pan from the heat, place one-sixth of the filling in the center of each tortilla, and roll the tortillas into burritos before serving.

Per Serving

calories: 535 | fat: 8g | carbs: 95g | protein: 29g | fiber: 21g

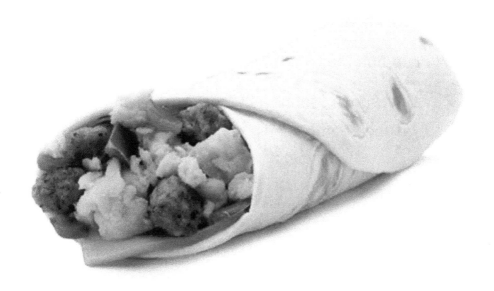

Breakfast Hummus Toast

Cook time: 5 minutes

Servings: 1

Ingredients

1 slice wheat bread, sprouted, toasted

¼ cup hummus

1 tablespoon sunflower seeds, unsalted, roasted 1 tablespoon hemp seeds

Instructions

1. Top the toasted bread with hummus, sunflower seeds, and hemp seeds. Enjoy!

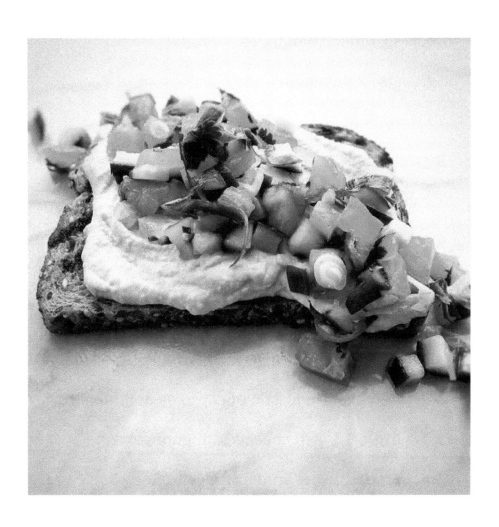

Dairy-Free Coconut Yogurt

Preparation Time: 5 minutes

Cooking Time: 10 minutes

Servings: 2 servings

Ingredients:

1 can coconut milk

4 vegan probiotic capsules

Directions:

1.   Shake coconut milk with a whole tube.

2.   Remove the plastic of capsules and mix in.

3.   Cut a 12-inch cheesecloth until stirred.

4.   Freeze or eat immediately.

Nutrition: Calories: 219 Fat: 10.1g Carbohydrates: 1.5g Protein: 7.9g

Vegan Green Avocado Smoothie

Preparation Time: 5 minutes

Cooking Time: 10 minutes

Servings: 2 servings

 Ingredients:

1 banana

1 cup water 1/2 avocado

1/2 lemon juice

1/2 cup coconut yogurt

Directions:

1.   Blend all Ingredients: until smooth.

Nutrition: Calories: 299 Fat: 1.1g Carbohydrates: 1.5g
Protein: 7.9g

Peach & Chia Seed Breakfast Parfait

Preparation Time: 5 minutes

Cooking Time: 10 minutes

Servings: 4

Ingredients:

¼ cup chia seeds

1 tablespoon pure maple syrup 1 cup of coconut milk

1 teaspoon ground cinnamon

3 medium peaches, diced small 2/3 cup granola

Directions:

1.   Find a small bowl and add the chia seeds, maple syrup, and coconut milk.

2.   Stir well, then cover and pop into the fridge for at least one hour.

3.   Find another bowl, add the peaches and sprinkle with the cinnamon. Pop to one side.

4. When it's time to serve, take two glasses and pour the chia mixture between the two.

5. Sprinkle the granola over the top, keeping a tiny amount to one side to use to decorate later.

6. Top with the peaches and the reserved granola and serve.

Nutrition:

Calories: 260 Fat: 13g Carbs: 22g Protein: 6g

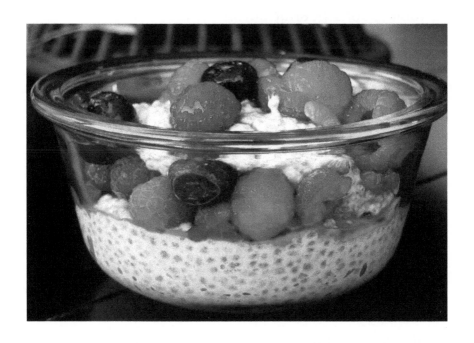

Buttered Overnight Oats

Cook time: 5 minutes

Servings: 1

Ingredients

¾ cup rolled oats

½ teaspoon cinnamon

1 tablespoon chia seeds 1 ripe banana, mashed

2 tablespoons peanut butter

½ cup + 1 tbsp. water

1 cup vanilla almond milk, unsweetened 2 tablespoons maple syrup

1 pinch salt

Instructions

1.   Get a mason jar and add oats, cinnamon, chia seeds, and salt to it. Combine properly. Stir in almond milk, mashed banana, and ½ cup water.

2.   Mix peanut butter and 1 tablespoon water in a bowl, then add into the jar and stir. Stir in the maple syrup and refrigerate overnight. Serve.

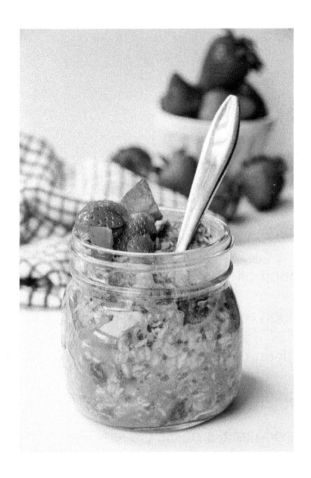

Protein Breakfast Burrito

Cook time: 30 minutes

Servings: 4

Ingredients

For tofu:

1 package (12 oz.) firm tofu

¼ cup parsley, minced

1 tablespoon hummus

1 teaspoon oil

1 teaspoon nutritional yeast

½ teaspoon cumin

½ teaspoon chili powder

¼ teaspoon salt 3 garlic cloves

For vegetables:

5 baby potatoes, sliced into pieces 2 cups kale, chopped

1 tablespoon water

1 medium red bell pepper, sliced thin

½ teaspoon ground cumin

½ teaspoon chili powder 1 pinch salt

For assembling:

4 large tortillas

1 medium avocado, ripe, chopped Hot sauce Cilantro

Instructions

1.   Preheat the oven to 400 F.

2.   Squeeze out excess moisture from tofu by wrapping it in a towel and placing a heavy object on top. Crumble into fine pieces and set aside.

3.   Place potatoes and red pepper onto a parchment paper-lined baking sheet, then sprinkle with water, cumin, chili powder, and salt. Toss and bake for 22

minutes. In the 17 minutes mark, add kale, toss and bake for extra 5 minutes.

4.   Preheat a skillet over medium heat. Add oil, garlic, and tofu once the skillet is hot, then sauté for 8 minutes, stirring frequently.

5.   Meanwhile, mix hummus, yeast, chili powder, cumin, and salt in a bowl, then add 2 tablespoons of water. Stir in parsley. Pour the mixture into the tofu and cook until slightly browned. Place aside.

6.   Roll out each tortilla and scoop a large portion of potato mixture, tofu mixture, avocado, cilantro, and a bit of hot sauce into the middle of each tortilla. Roll up and seal the seam, then serve immediately.

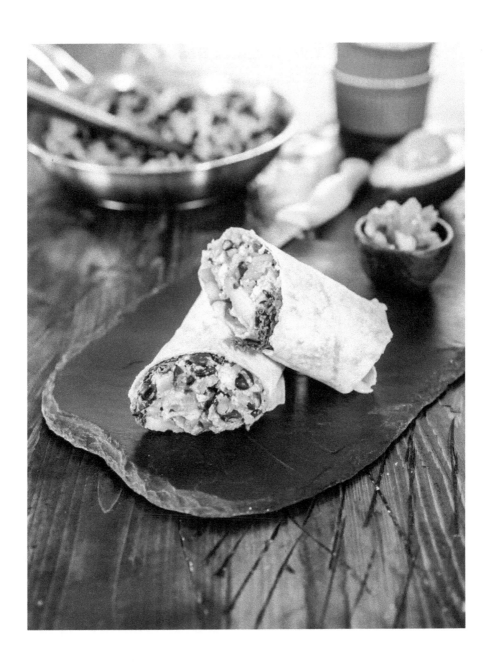

Avocado Toast with White Beans

Preparation Time: 5 minutes

Cooking Time: 6 minutes

Servings: 4

Ingredients:

½ cup canned white beans, 2 tsp tahini paste

2 teaspoons lemon juice

½ teaspoon salt

½ avocado, peeled and pit removed 4 slices whole-grain bread, toasted

½ cup grape tomatoes, cut in half

Directions:

1.   Grab a small bowl and add the beans, tahini, ½ lemon juice, and ½ salt. Mash with a fork.

2.   Take another bowl and add the avocado and the remaining lemon juice and salt. Mash together.

3.　　Place your toast onto a flat surface and add the mashed beans, spreading well.

4.　　Top with the avocado and the sliced tomatoes, then serve and enjoy.

Nutrition:

Calories: 140 Fat: 5g Carbs: 13g Protein: 5g

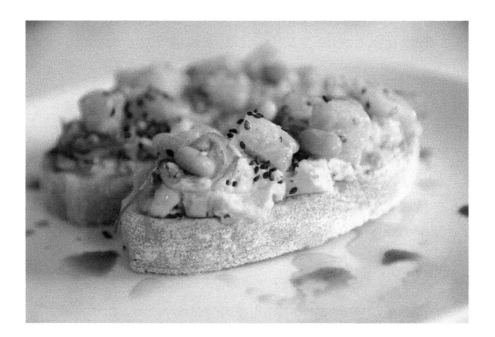

Gingerbread Waffles

Preparation Time: 30 minutes

Cooking Time: 20 minutes

Servings: 6

Ingredients:

1 cup spelled flour

2 teaspoon baking powder

¼ teaspoon salt

1 tbsp flax seeds 1 ½ tsp cinnamon 2 tsp ground ginger

4 tablespoon coconut sugar

¼ teaspoon baking soda 1½ tablespoon olive oil 1 cup non-dairy milk

1 tbsp apple vinegar 2 tbsp molasses

Directions:

1. Take a waffle iron, oil generously, and preheat.

2. Take a large bowl and add the dry ingredients. Stir well together.

3. Put the wet ingredients into another bowl and stir until combined.

4. Stir the dry and wet together until combined.

5. Pour the mixture into the waffle iron and cook at a medium temperature for 20 minutes.

6. Open carefully and remove.

7. Serve and enjoy.

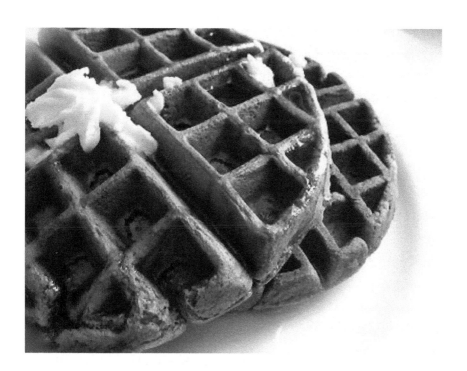

Greek Garbanzo Beans on Toast

Preparation Time: 25 minutes

Cooking Time: 5 minutes

Servings: 2

Ingredients:

2 tablespoons olive oil

3 small shallots, finely diced

2 large garlic cloves, finely diced

¼ teaspoon smoked paprika

½ teaspoon sweet paprika

½ teaspoon cinnamon

½ teaspoon salt

½-1 teaspoon sugar, to taste Black pepper, to taste

1 x 14 oz. can peel plum tomatoes 2 cups cooked garbanzo beans

5-6 slices of crusty bread, fresh parsley, and dill

Pitted Kalamata olives

Directions:

1.   Pop a skillet over medium heat and add the oil.

2.   Put the shallots in the pan and let them cook for six minutes.

3.   Add the garlic and cook until ready, then add the other spices to the pan.

4.   Stir well, then add the tomatoes.

5.   Simmer until the sauce thickens.

6.   Add the garbanzo beans and warm through.

7.   Season with sugar, salt, and pepper, then serve and enjoy.

Nutrition: calories 709 fat 12 carbs 23 protein 19

Easy Hummus Toast

Preparation Time: 10 minutes

Cooking Time: 10 minutes

Servings: 1

Ingredients:

1 slice sprouted wheat bread

¼ cup hummus

1 tablespoon hemp seeds

1 tablespoon roasted unsalted sunflower seeds

Directions:

1.   Start by toasting your bread.

2.   Top with the hummus and seeds, then eat!

Nutrition:

calories 316 fat 16 carbs 13 protein 18

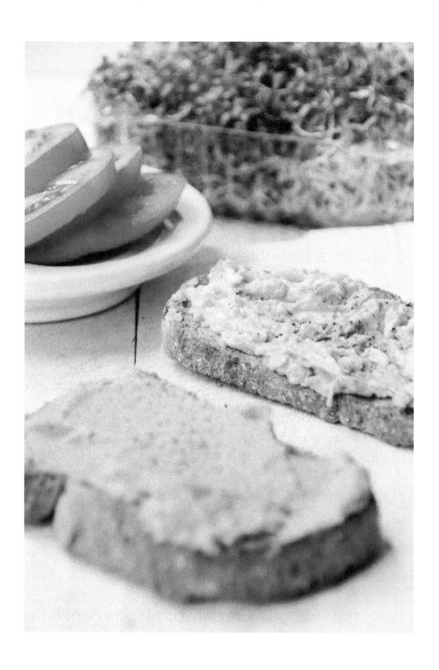

Chickpea Scramble Breakfast Basin

Cook time: 10 minutes

Servings: 2

Ingredients

For chickpea scramble:

1   can (15 oz.) chickpeas A drizzle olive oil

¼ white onion, diced

2   garlic cloves, minced

½ teaspoon turmeric

½ teaspoon pepper

½ teaspoon salt

For breakfast basin:

1 avocado, wedged Greens, combined Handful parsley, minced Handful cilantro, minced

Instructions

For chickpea scramble:

1.   Scoop out the chickpeas and a little bit of its water into a bowl. Slightly mash the chickpeas using a fork, intentionally omitting some. Stir in the turmeric, pepper, and salt until adequately combined.

2.   Sauté onions in extra-virgin olive oil, then add garlic and cook for 1 minute. Stir in the chickpeas and sauté for 5 minutes.

For breakfast basin and serving:

1.   Get 2 breakfast basins. Layer the bottom of the basins with the combined greens. Top with chickpea scramble, parsley, and cilantro. Enjoy with avocado wedges.

Brown Rice Breakfast Pudding

Preparation Time: 5 minutes

Cooking Time: 15 minutes

Servings: 4 servings

Ingredients:

2 cups almond milk

1 cup dates (chopped) 1 apple (chopped) Salt to taste

1/4 cup almonds (toasted) 1 cinnamon stick

Ground cloves to taste 3 cups cooked rice

1 tablespoon raisins

Directions:

1.   Mix the rice, milk, cinnamon stick, spices, and dates in a small saucepan and steam when the paste is heavy.

2.   Take the cinnamon stick down. Stir in the fruit, raisins, salt, and blend.

3.   Serve with almonds bread.

Nutrition: Calories: 299 Fat: 1.1g Carbohydrates: 71.5g
Protein: 7.9g

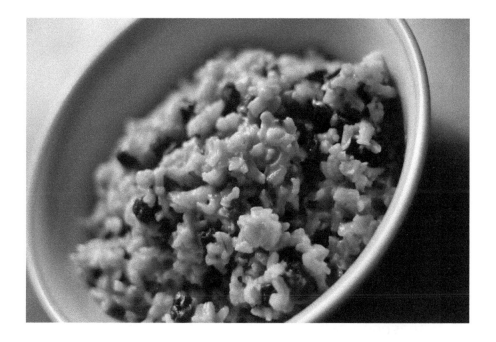

Chickpea Scramble Breakfast Basin

Cook time: 10 minutes

Servings: 2

Ingredients

For chickpea scramble:

1 can (15 oz.) chickpeas A drizzle olive oil

¼ white onion, diced

2 garlic cloves, minced

½ teaspoon turmeric

½ teaspoon pepper

½ teaspoon salt

For breakfast basin:

1 avocado, wedged Greens, combined Handful parsley, minced Handful cilantro, minced

Instructions

For chickpea scramble:

1.   Scoop out the chickpeas and a little bit of its water into a bowl. Slightly mash the chickpeas using a fork, intentionally omitting some. Stir in the turmeric, pepper, and salt until adequately combined.

2.   Add garlic to the sautéed onions and cook for 1 minute. Stir in the chickpeas and sauté for 5 minutes.

For breakfast basin and serving:

1.   Get 2 breakfast basins. Layer the bottom of the basins with the combined greens. Top with chickpea scramble, parsley, and cilantro. Enjoy with avocado wedges.

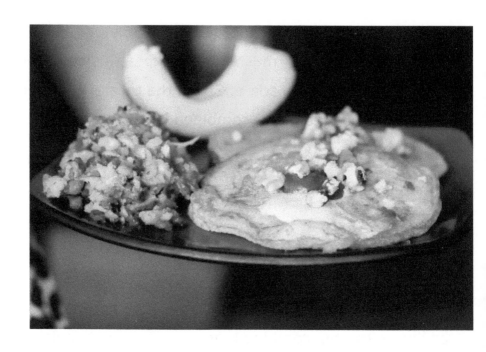

Quinoa, Oats, Hazelnut and Blueberry Salad

Cook time: 35 minutes

Servings: 8

Ingredients

1 cup golden quinoa, dry 1 cup oats, cut into pieces 2 cups blueberries

2 cups hazelnuts, roughly chopped, toasted

½ cup dry millet

2 large lemons, zested, juiced 3 tablespoons olive oil, divided

½ cup maple syrup 1 cup Greek yogurt

1 (1-inch) piece fresh ginger, peeled, cut

¼ teaspoon nutmeg

Instructions

1.   Combine quinoa, oats, and millet in a large bowl. Rinse, drain and set aside.

2.   Add one tablespoon olive oil into a saucepan and place over medium-high heat. Cook the rinsed grains in it for 3 minutes. Add 4 ½ cups water and salt. Add the zest of 1 lemon and ginger.

3.   When the mixture boils, cover the pot and cook in reduced heat for 20 minutes. Remove from heat. Let rest for 5 minutes. Uncover and fluff with a fork. Discard the ginger and layer the grains on a large baking sheet. Let cool for 30 minutes.

4.   Transfer the grains into a large bowl and mix in the remaining lemon zest.

5.   Combine the juice of both lemons with the remaining olive oil in a separate bowl. Stir in the yogurt, maple syrup, and nutmeg. Pour the mixture into the grains and stir. Mix in the blueberries and hazelnuts. Refrigerate overnight, then serve.

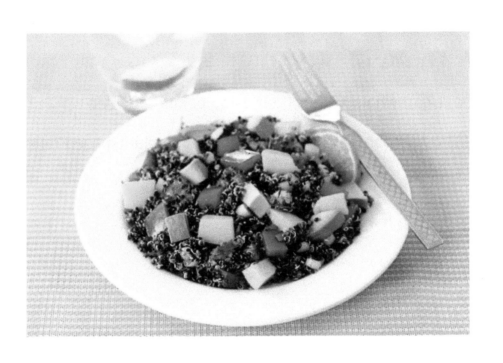

Applesauce Pancakes

Prep time: 5 minutes

Cook time: 15 minutes

Makes 8 pancakes

Ingredients:

1 cup whole-wheat flour 1 tsp baking powder

½ teaspoon ground cinnamon 1 cup plant-based milk

½ cup unsweetened applesauce

¼ cup maple syrup

1 teaspoon vanilla extract

Directions:

1.   Put together cinnamon, flour and baking powder in a large bowl.

2.   Stir in the milk, applesauce, maple syrup, and vanilla until no dry flour is left and the batter is smooth.

3.　For each pancake, pour ¼ cup of batter onto the hot skillet. Once bubbles form over the top of the pancake and the sides begin to brown and flip.

4.　Repeat until all of the batters are used and serve.

Nutrition:

per Serving (2 pancakes) calories: 210 | fat: 2g | carbs: 44g | protein: 5g | fiber: 5g

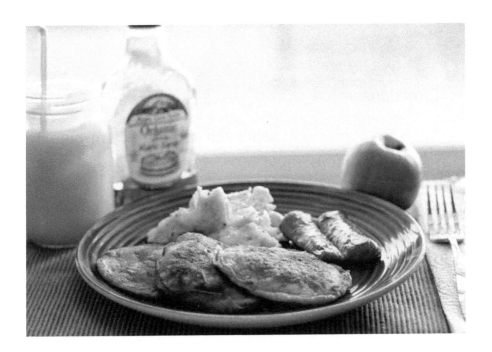

Chocolate Peanut Butter Quinoa

Prep time: 5 minutes

Cook time: 10 minutes

Serves 2

Ingredients:

1 cup plant-based milk 2 cups cooked quinoa

1 tablespoon maple syrup 1 tablespoon cocoa powder

1 tablespoon defatted peanut powder

Directions:

1.   In a medium saucepan over medium-high heat, bring the milk to a boil.

2. Stir in the quinoa, maple syrup, cocoa powder, and peanut powder when boiling.

3.   Cook, uncovered, for 5 minutes, stirring every other minute. Serve warm.

Nutrition:

Per Serving calories: 339 | fat: 8g | carbs: 53g | protein: 14g | fiber: 7g

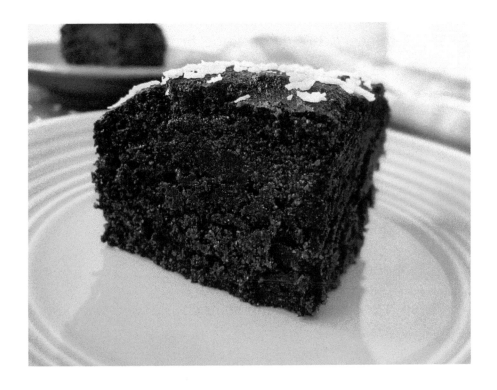

Tofu and Vegetable Breakfast Scramble

Prep time: 5 minutes

Cook time: 15 minutes

Serves 2

Ingredients:

1 (14-ounce / 397-g) package firm or extra-firm tofu 4 ounces (113 g) mushrooms, sliced

½ bell pepper, diced

2 tablespoons nutritional yeast

1 tablespoon vegetable broth or water

½ teaspoon garlic powder

½ teaspoon onion powder

⅛ tsp black pepper 1 cup spinach

Directions:

1.   Heat a large skillet over medium-low heat.

2.   Drain the tofu, then place it in the skillet and mash it down with a fork or mixing spoon. Stir in the

mushrooms, bell pepper, nutritional yeast, broth, garlic powder, onion powder, and pepper. Let it cook for 10 minutes, stirring once after about 5 minutes.

3.   Uncover and stir in the spinach. Serve.

Nutrition:

Per Serving calories: 230 | fat: 10g | carbs: 16g | protein: 27g | fiber: 7g

Peach & Chia Seed Breakfast Parfait

Preparation Time: 5 minutes

Cooking Time: 10 minutes

Servings: 4

Ingredients:

¼ cup chia seeds

1 tablespoon pure maple syrup 1 cup of coconut milk

1 teaspoon ground cinnamon

3 medium peaches, diced small 2/3 cup granola

Directions:

1.   Find a small bowl and add the chia seeds, maple syrup, and coconut milk.

2.   Stir well, then cover and pop into the fridge for at least one hour.

3.   Find another bowl, add the peaches and sprinkle with the cinnamon. Pop to one side.

4.   When it's time to serve, take two glasses and pour the chia mixture between the two.

5.   Sprinkle the granola over the top, keeping a tiny amount to one side to use to decorate later.

6.   Top with the peaches and the reserved granola and serve.

Nutrition: calories 260 fat 13 carbs 22 protein 6

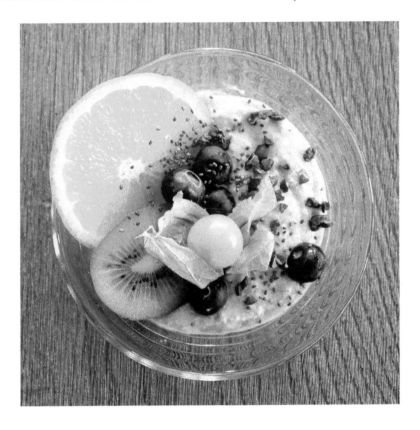

Avocado Toast with Black Beans

Preparation Time: 5 minutes

Cooking Time: 6 minutes

Servings: 4

Ingredients:

½ cup beans 2 tsp tahini paste

2 tsp lemon juice

½ teaspoon salt

½ avocado, peeled and pit removed 4 slices whole-grain bread, toasted

½ cup grape tomatoes, cut in half

Directions:

1.   Grab a small bowl and add the beans, tahini, ½ lemon juice, and ½ salt. Mash with a fork.

2.   Take another bowl and add the avocado and the remaining lemon juice and salt. Mash together.

3.   Place your toast onto a flat surface and add the mashed beans, spreading well.

4.   Top with the avocado and the sliced tomatoes, then serve and enjoy.

Nutrition: calories 140 fat 5 carbs 13 protein 5

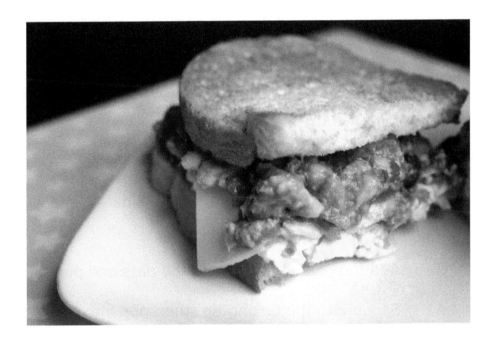

Oatmeal & Peanut Butter Breakfast Bar

Preparation Time: 10 minutes

Cooking Time: 0 minutes

Servings: 8

Ingredients:

1 ½ cups date, pit removed

½ cup peanut butter

½ cup old-fashioned rolled oats

Directions:

1.   Grease a baking tin and pop to one side.

2.   Grab your food processor, add the dates, and whizz until chopped.

3.   Add the peanut butter and the oats and pulse.

4.   Scoop into the baking tin, then pop into the fridge or freezer until set.

5.   Serve and enjoy.

Nutrition: calories 232 fat 9 carbs 32 protein 8

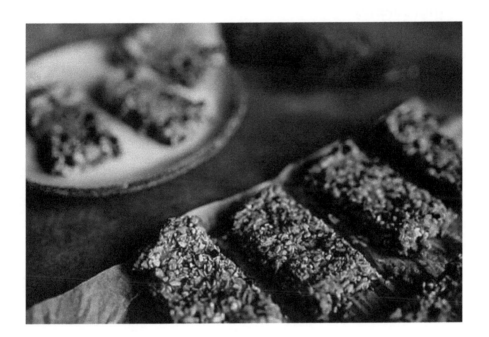

Chocolate Chip Coconut Pancakes

Preparation Time: 5 minutes

Cooking Time: 30 minutes

Servings: 8 servings

Ingredients:

11/4 cup oats

1 teaspoon coconut flakes 2 cup plant milk

11/4 cup maple syrup

11/3 cup of chocolate chips 2 1/4 cups buckwheat flour 2 teaspoon baking powder 1 teaspoon vanilla essence 2 teaspoon flaxseed meal Salt (optional)

Directions:

1.   Put the flaxseed and cook over medium heat until the paste becomes a little moist.

2.   Remove seeds.

3.   Stir the buckwheat, oats, coconut chips, baking powder, and salt with each other in a wide dish.

4.   In a large dish, stir together the retained flax water with the sugar, maple syrup, vanilla essence.

5.   Put together the wet ingredients with the dry ones and shake to combine

6.   Place over medium heat the non-stick grill pan.

7.   Pour 1/4 cup flour onto the grill pan with each pancake, and scatter gently.

8.   Cook for five to six minutes before the pancakes appear somewhat crispy.

Nutrition:

Calories: 198 Fat: 9.1g Carbs: 11.5g Protein: 7.9g

Apple-Lemon Bowl

Preparation Time: 5 minutes

Cooking Time: 15 minutes

Servings: 1-2 servings

Ingredients:

6 apples

3 tablespoons walnuts

7 dates Lemon juice

1/2 teaspoon cinnamon

Directions:

1.   Root the apples, then break them into wide bits.

2.   In a food cup, put seeds, part of the lime juice, almonds, spices, and three-quarters of the apples. Thinly slice until finely ground.

3.   Apply the remaining apples and lemon juice and make slices.

Nutrition:

Calories: 249 Fat: 5.1g Carbs: 71.5g Protein: 7.9g

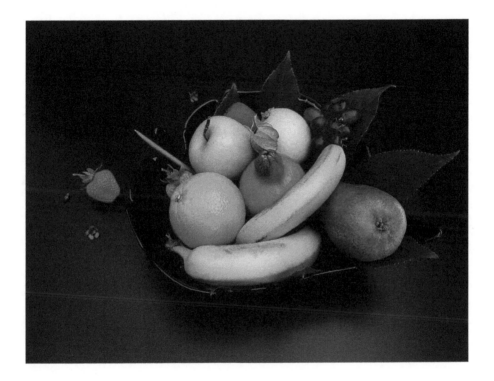

Breakfast Scramble

Preparation Time: 15 minutes

Cooking Time: 35 minutes

Servings: 6 servings

Ingredients:

1 red onion

2 tablespoons soy sauce 2 cups sliced mushrooms Salt to taste

11/2 teaspoon black pepper 11/2 teaspoons turmeric 1/4 teaspoon cayenne

3 cloves garlic

1 red bell pepper

1 large head cauliflower 1 green bell pepper

Directions:

1.   In a small pan, put all vegetables and cook until crispy.

2.　　Stir in the cauliflower and cook for four to six minutes or until it smooth.

3.　　Add spices to the pan and cook for another five minutes.

Nutrition:

Calories: 199 Fat: 1.1g Carbs: 14.5g Protein: 7.9g

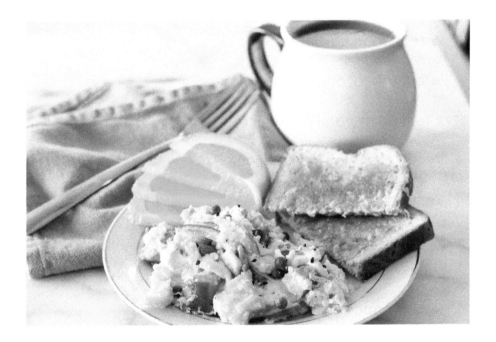

No-Bake Chewy Granola Bars

Preparation Time: 10 minutes

Cooking Time: 10 minutes

Servings: 8

Ingredients:

¼ teaspoon cinnamon

¼ teaspoon salt

½ teaspoon cardamom

¼ cup of coconut oil 1 cup oats

1 teaspoon vanilla extract

½ cup raw almonds, sliced

¼ cup sunflower seeds

½ cup pumpkin seeds 1¼ teaspoon nutmeg 1 tbsp chia seeds

¼ cup honey

1 cup dried figs, chopped

Directions:

1.   Pop to one side of a baking dish.

2.   Grab a saucepan and add salt, honey, oil, and spices.

3.   Pop over medium heat and stir until it melts together.

4.   Decrease the heat, add the oats, and stir.

5.   Add the dried fruit, seeds, and nuts, and stir through again.

6.   Cook for 10 minutes.

7.   Take off the heat and move the oat mixture to the pan.

8.   Press down until it's packed firm.

9.   Let it cool, then cut into 8 bars.

10.   Serve and enjoy.

Nutrition: calories 308 fat 14 carbs 35 protein 6

Tasty Oatmeal and Carrot Cake

Preparation Time: 5 minutes

Cooking Time: 10 minutes

Servings: 2

Ingredients:

1 cup of water

½ teaspoon of cinnamon 1 cup of rolled oats

Salt

¼ cup of raisins

½ cup of shredded carrots 1 cup of non-dairy milk

¼ teaspoon of allspice

Toppings:

½ teaspoon of vanilla extract

¼ cup of chopped walnuts

2 tablespoons of maple syrup

2 tablespoons of shredded coconut

Directions:

1. Bring the non-dairy milk, oats, and water to a simmer.

2. Now, add the carrots, vanilla extract, raisins, salt, cinnamon, and allspice. You need to simmer all the ingredients, but do not forget to stir them. You will know that they are ready when the liquid is fully absorbed into all the ingredients (in about 7-10 minutes).

3. Transfer the thickened dish to bowls. You can top them with coconut or walnuts.

4. This nutritious bowl will allow you to kickstart your day.

Nutrition: calories 210 fat 11 carbs 42 protein 4

Almond Butter Banana Overnight Oats

Preparation Time: 5 minutes

Cooking Time: 10 minutes

Servings: 2

Ingredients:

½ cup rolled oats 1 cup almond milk

1 tablespoon chia seeds

¼ teaspoon vanilla extract

½ teaspoon ground cinnamon

1 tbspoon honey or maple syrup 1 banana, sliced

2 tablespoons natural almond butter

Directions:

1.   Put together the oats, milk, chia seeds, vanilla, cinnamon, and honey in a small bowl.

2.   Stir to combine, then divide half of the mixture between two bowls.

3.   Top with the banana and peanut butter, then add the remaining mixture.

4.   Cover, then pop into the fridge overnight.

5.   Serve and enjoy.

Nutrition: calories 227 fat 11 carbs 35 protein 7

Chocolate Chip Banana Pancake

Preparation Time: 15 minutes

Cooking Time: 3 minutes

Servings: 6

Ingredients:

1 banana 2 tbsp coconut sugar

3 tablespoons coconut oil, melted 1 cup of coconut milk

1 ½ cups flour 1 teaspoon baking soda

½ cup vegan chocolate chips Olive oil, for frying

Directions:

1.   Grab a large bowl and add the banana, sugar, oil, and milk. Stir well.

2.   Add the flour and baking soda and stir again until combined.

3.   Add the chocolate chips and fold through, then pop to one side.

4.   Put a skillet over medium heat and add a drop of oil.

5.   Pour ¼ of the batter into the pan and move the pan to cover.

6.   Cook for 3 minutes, then flip and cook on the other side.

7.   Repeat with the remaining pancakes, then serve and enjoy.

Nutrition:

Calories: 105 Fat: 13g Carbs: 23g Protein: 5g

Avocado and 'Sausage' Breakfast Sandwich

Preparation Time: 15 minutes

Cooking Time: 10 minutes

Servings: 1

Ingredients:

1   vegan sausage patty 1 cup kale, chopped

2   teaspoons extra-virgin olive oil 1 tablespoon pepitas

Salt and pepper, to taste

1 tablespoon vegan mayo

1/8 teaspoon chipotle powder 1 teaspoon jalapeno chopped 1 English muffin, toasted

¼ avocado, sliced

Directions:

1.   Place a sauté pan over high heat and add a drop of oil.

2.   Add the vegan patty and cook for 2 minutes.

3.   Flip the patty, then add the kale and pepitas.

4.   Season well, then cook for another few minutes until the patty is cooked.

5.   Find a small bowl and add the mayo, chipotle powder, and jalapeno. Stir well to combine.

6.   Place the muffin onto a flat surface, spread with the spicy mayo, then top with the patty.

7.   Add the sliced avocado, then serve and enjoy.

Nutrition:

Calories: 573 Fat: 23g Carbs: 36g Protein: 21g

Cinnamon Rolls with Cashew Frosting

Preparation Time: 25 minutes

Cooking Time: 25 minutes

Servings: 12

Ingredients:

3 tablespoons vegan butter

¾ cup unsweetened almond milk

½ teaspoon salt

3 tablespoons sugar 1 teaspoon vanilla extract

½ cup pumpkin puree

3 cups all-purpose flour

2 ¼ teaspoons dried active yeast

3 tablespoons softened vegan butter 3 tablespoons brown sugar

½ teaspoon cinnamon

½ cup cashews

½ cup icing sugar

2 tsp vanilla extract 1 cup almond milk

Directions:

1.   Soak the cashews for 1 hour in boiling water.

2.   Grease a baking sheet and pop to one side.

3.   Find a small bowl, add the butter, and pop into the microwave to melt.

4.   Add the sugar and stir well, then set aside to cool.

5.   Grab a large bowl and add the flour, salt, and yeast. Stir well to mix.

6.   Place the cooled butter into a jug, add the pumpkin puree, vanilla, and almond milk. Stir well together.

7.   Put together the wet ingredients and the dry ones, then stir well to combine.

8.   Tip onto a flat surface and knead for 5 minutes, adding extra flour as needed to avoid sticking.

9.   Pop back into the bowl, cover with plastic wrap, and pop into the fridge overnight.

10.   Take the dough off the fridge and spread with your fingers.

11.   Roll with a rolling pin to obtain a 18" rectangle, then spread with butter.

12.   Find a small bowl and add the sugar and cinnamon. Mix well, then sprinkle with the butter.

13.   Roll the dough into a large sausage, then slice into sections.

14.   Place onto the greased baking sheet and leave in a dark place to rise for one hour.

15.   Preheat the oven to 350°F.

16.   Put the drained cashews in your blender. Whizz until smooth.

17.   Add the sugar and the vanilla, then whizz again.

Nutrition: Calories: 243 Fat: 9g Carbs: 34g Protein: 4g

18.   Add the almond milk until it reaches your desired consistency.

19.   Pop into the oven and bake for 20 minutes until golden.

20.   Pour the glaze over the top, then serve and enjoy.

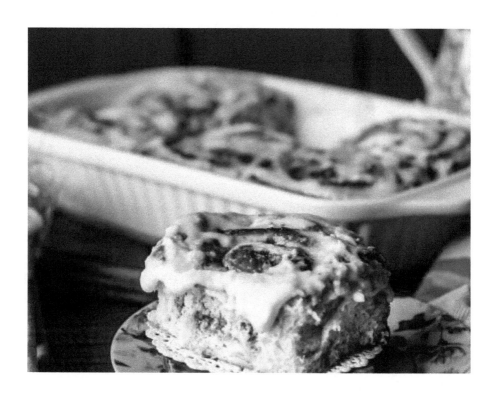

Breakfast Scramble

Preparation Time: 10 minutes

Cooking Time: 30 minutes

Servings: 6 servings

Ingredients:

1 red onion

2 tablespoons soy sauce 2 cups sliced mushrooms Salt to taste

11/2 teaspoon black pepper 11/2 teaspoons turmeric 1/4 teaspoon cayenne

3 cloves garlic

1 red bell pepper

1 large head cauliflower 1 green bell pepper

Directions:

1.   In a small pan, put all vegetables and cook until crispy.

2.   Stir in the cauliflower and cook for four to six minutes or until it smooth.

3.   Add spices to the pan and cook for another five minutes.

Nutrition: Calories: 199 Fat: 1.1g Carbohydrates: 14.5g Protein: 7.9g

Potato Fried Rice Breakfast

Prep time: 15 minutes

Cook time: 12 minutes

Serves 4

Ingredients:

1 onion 1 stalk celery

$1/3$ cup chopped green bell pepper

½ cup water

2 large boiled potatoes, peeled or unpeeled, and chopped
1 cup cooked brown rice

1 teaspoon ground cumin 1 tablespoon soy sauce

Directions:

1.   Sauté the onion, celery, and green pepper in ¼ cup of the water in a large non-stick frying pan for 5 minutes.

2.   Add the potatoes and the remaining ¼ cup water. Cook, stirring gently, until the vegetables are tender, about 5 minutes. Stir in the rice, cumin, and soy sauce.

Cook, stirring, until the bottom browns lightly, about 2 minutes.

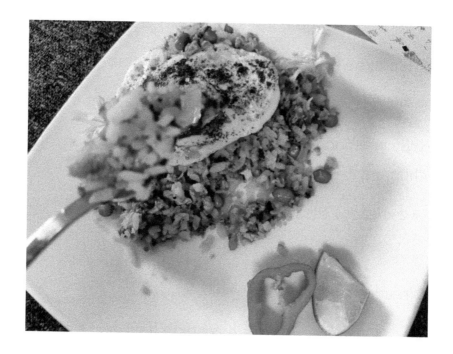

Avocado and 'Sausage' Breakfast Sandwich

Preparation Time: 15 minutes

Cooking Time: 10 minutes

Servings: 1

Ingredients:

1 vegan sausage patty 1 cup kale, chopped

2 tsp extra-virgin olive oil 1 tbsp pepitas

Salt and pepper, to taste 1 tablespoon vegan mayo

1/8 teaspoon chipotle powder 1 teaspoon jalapeno chopped 1 English muffin, toasted

¼ avocado, sliced

Directions:

1.   Place a sauté pan over high heat and add a drop of oil.

2.   Add the vegan patty and cook for 2 minutes.

3.   Flip the patty then add the kale and pepitas.

4.   Season well then cook for another few minutes until the patty is cooked.

5.   Find a small bowl and add the mayo, chipotle powder, and jalapeno. Stir well to combine.

6.   Place the muffin onto a flat surface, spread with the spicy mayo then top with the patty.

7.   Add the sliced avocado then serve and enjoy.

Nutrition: calories 573 fat 23 carbs 36 protein 21

Cinnamon Rolls with Cashew Frosting

Preparation Time: 25 minutes

Cooking Time: 25 minutes

Servings: 12

Ingredients:

3 tablespoons vegan butter

¾ cup unsweetened almond milk

½ teaspoon salt

4 tbsp caster sugar 1 teaspoon vanilla extract

½ cup pumpkin puree

3 cups all-purpose flour

2 ¼ teaspoons dried active yeast

3 tablespoons softened vegan butter 3 tablespoons brown sugar

½ teaspoon cinnamon

½ cup cashews

½ cup icing sugar

2 tsp vanilla extract 1 cup almond milk

Directions:

1.　Soak the cashews for 1 hour in boiling water.

2.　Grease a baking sheet and pop to one side.

3.　Find a small bowl, add the butter, and pop into the microwave to melt.

4.　Add the sugar and stir well, then set aside to cool.

5.　Grab a large bowl and add the flour, salt, and yeast. Stir well to mix.

6.　Place the cooled butter into a jug, add the pumpkin puree, vanilla, and almond milk. Stir well together.

7.　Put together the dry ingredients with the wet ones and stir well to combine.

8.　Tip onto a flat surface and knead for 5 minutes, adding extra flour as needed to avoid sticking.

9.　Pop back into the bowl, cover with plastic wrap, and pop into the fridge overnight.

10.　Shape with your fingers.

11. Spread with butter.

12. Find a small bowl and add the sugar and cinnamon. Mix well, then sprinkle with the butter.

13. Roll the dough into a large sausage then slice into sections.

14. Place onto the greased baking sheet and leave in a dark place to rise for one hour.

15. Preheat the oven to 350°F.

16. Put the drained cashews in your blender. Whizz until smooth.

17. Add the sugar and the vanilla, then whizz again.

18. Add the almond milk until it reaches your desired consistency.

19. Bake for 25 minutes.

20. Pour the glaze over the top, then serve and enjoy.

Nutrition: calories 243 fat 9 carbs 34 protein 4

Vegan Variety Poppy Seed Scones

Preparation Time: 5 minutes

Cooking Time: 10 minutes

Servings: 12.

Ingredients:

1 cup white sugar 2 cups flour

Juice from 1 lemon Zest

4 teaspoon baking powder

½ teaspoon salt

1 cup Earth Balance or vegan butter

2 tablespoon poppy seeds

½ cup soymilk 1/3 cup water

Directions:

1.   Heat the oven to 400 degrees Fahrenheit.

2.   Next, mix the sugar, the flour, the powder, and the salt in a big mixing bowl. Add the vegan butter to the mixture and cut it up until you create a sand-like mixture.

Next, add the lemon juice, the lemon zest, and the poppy seeds. Add the water and the soy milk, and stir the ingredients well.

3.   Portion the batter out over a baking sheet in about ¼ cup portions. Allow the scones to bake for fifteen minutes and let them cool before serving. Enjoy.

Nutrition: calories 205 fat 3 carbs 12 protein 6

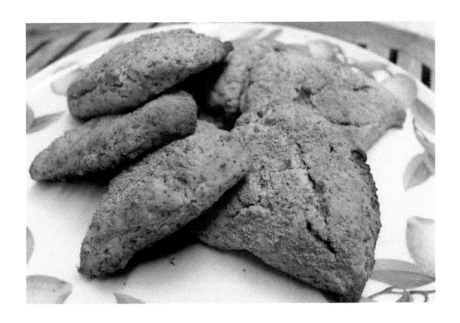

Sweet Pomegranate Porridge

Preparation Time: 5 minutes

Cooking Time: 20 minutes

Servings: 4

Ingredients:

2 Cups Oats

1 ½ Cups Water

1 ½ Cups Pomegranate Juice

2 Tablespoons Pomegranate Molasses

Directions:

1.   Mix well all the ingredients.

2.   Seal the lid, and cook on high pressure for four minutes.

3.   Use a quick release, and serve warm.

Nutrition: calories 177 fat 6 carbs 23 protein 8

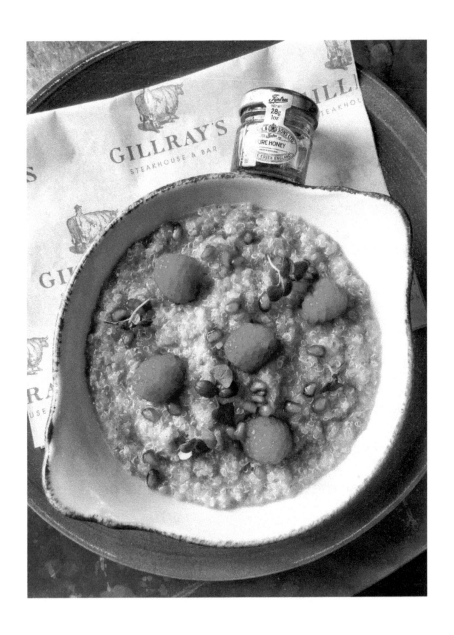

Apple Oatmeal

Preparation Time: 5 minutes

Cooking Time: 20 minutes

Servings: 4

Ingredients:

¼ Teaspoon Sea Salt 1 Cup Cashew Milk

1   Cup Strawberries, Halved & Fresh 1 Tablespoon Brown Sugar

2   Cups Apples, Diced 3 Cups Water

¼ Teaspoon Coconut Oil

½ Cup Steel Cut Oats

Directions:

1.   Start by greasing your instant pot with oil, and add everything to it except for the milk and berries.

2.   Allow for a natural pressure release, and then add in your milk and strawberries. Mix well, and serve warm.

Nutrition: calories 435 fat 7 carbs 34 protein 8

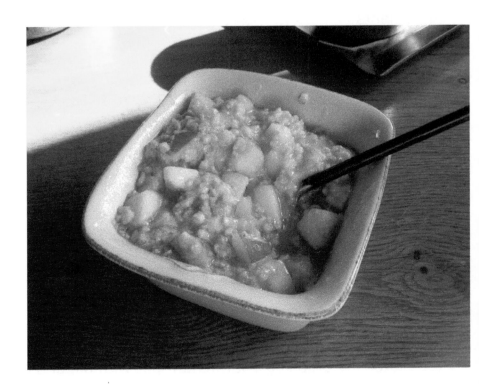

Black Bean and Sweet Potato Hash

Preparation Time: 10 minutes

Cooking Time: 30 minutes

Servings: 4 servings

Ingredients:

1 cup onion (chopped) 1/3 cup vegetable broth 2 garlic (minced)

1 cup cooked black beans

2 teaspoons hot chili powder

2 cups chopped sweet potatoes

Directions:

1.   Put the onions in a saucepan over medium heat and add the seasoning, and mix.

2.   Add potatoes and chili flakes, then mix.

3.   Cook for around 12 minutes more until the vegetables are cooked thoroughly.

4.   Add the green onion, beans, and salt

5. Cook for more 2 minutes and serve.

Nutrition:

Calories: 239 Fat: 1.1g Carbs: 71.5g Protein: 7.9g

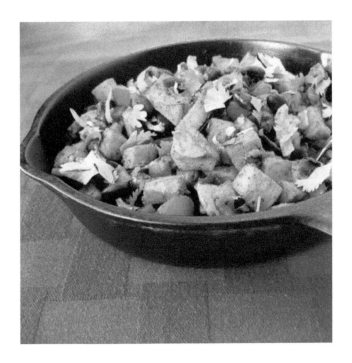

Apple-Walnut Breakfast Bread

Preparation Time: 15 minutes

Cooking Time: 60 minutes

Servings: 8 servings

Ingredients:

11/2 cups apple sauce 1/3 cup plant milk

2 cups all-purpose flour Salt to taste

1 teaspoon ground cinnamon

1 tablespoon flax seeds mixed with 2 tablespoons warm water 3/4 cup brown sugar

1 teaspoon baking powder 1/2 cup chopped walnuts

Directions:

1.   Preheat to 375°F.

2.   Combine the apple sauce, sugar, milk, and flax mixture in a jar and mix.

3.   Mix salt, cinnamon, baking powder and flour in a small bowl.

4.   Simply add dry ingredients into the wet ingredients and combine to make slices.

5.   Bake for 25 minutes until it becomes light brown.

Nutrition: Calories: 309 Fat: 9.1g Carbs: 16.5g Protein: 6.9g

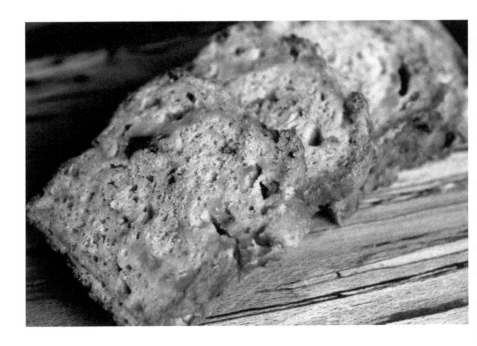

Breakfast Barley with Fruit

Prep time: 5 minutes

Cook time: 50 minutes

Serves 2

Ingredients

1 to 1½ cups orange juice 1 cup pearled barley

2 tablespoons dried currants

3 to 4 dried unsulfured apricots, chopped 1 small cinnamon stick

⅛ teaspoon ground cloves

Pinch salt, or to taste

Directions:

1.   Bring water and orange juice to a boil. Add the barley, salt, currants, apricots, cinnamon stick and cloves. Bring to boil and cook for 45 minutes. If the barley is not tender after 45 minutes, add up to an additional ½ cup of orange juice and cook for another 10 minutes.

2.   Remove the cinnamon stick before serving.

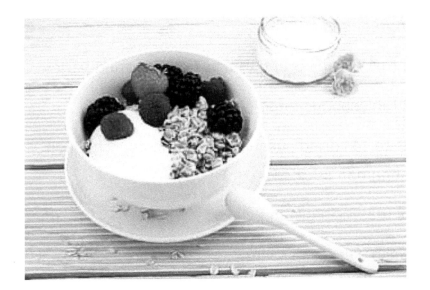

Breakfast Tofu Slices

Prep time: 10 minutes

Cook time: 30 minutes

Makes 12 slices

Ingredients:

2 (16-ounce / 454-g) packages sprouted or extra-firm tofu, drained 1 tablespoon reduced-sodium tamari

¼ cup nutritional yeast

1 teaspoon ground cumin

½ teaspoon garlic powder

½ teaspoon ground turmeric

½ teaspoon yellow curry powder

¼ teaspoon black pepper

Directions:

1.   Take the oven to 400ºF (205ºC). Line a baking sheet with parchment paper.

2.   Cut every tofu package in six pieces.

3.   Combine the spices in a food container.

4.   Place tofu on the baking sheet. Spread any extra seasoning mix on top. Bake for 30 minutes, flipping halfway through.

5.   Serve and enjoy!

Breakfast Cookies

Preparation Time: 10 minutes

Cooking Time: 6 minutes

Servings: 24-32

Ingredients:

Dry Ingredients:

½ teaspoon baking powder 2 cups rolled oats

½ teaspoon baking soda

Wet Ingredients:

1   teaspoon pure vanilla extract

2   eggs (2 tbsp ground flaxseed and around 6 tablespoons of water, mix and put aside for 15 minutes)

coconut oil (melted) maple syrup

½ cup natural creamy peanut butter 2 ripe bananas

Add-in Ingredients:

½ cup finely chopped walnuts

½ cup raisins Optional Topping:

2 tablespoons chopped walnuts 2 tablespoons raisins

Directions:

1.	Heat the oven up to 325°F, then use parchment paper to line a baking sheet and put it aside.

2.	Add the bananas, then use a fork to mash them until smooth. Add in the other wet ingredients and mix until well incorporated.

3.	Add the dry ingredients and then use a rubber spatula to stir and fold them into the dry ingredients until well mixed. Stir in the walnuts and raisins.

4.	Scoop the cookie dough making sure that you leave adequate space between the cookies.

5.	Let it cook into the oven for 15 minutes. Once ready, let the cookies cool on the baking sheet for around 10 minutes.

6.	Lift the cookies carefully from the baking sheet onto a cooling rack to further cool.

Nutrition: calories 565 fat 6 carbs 32 protein 8

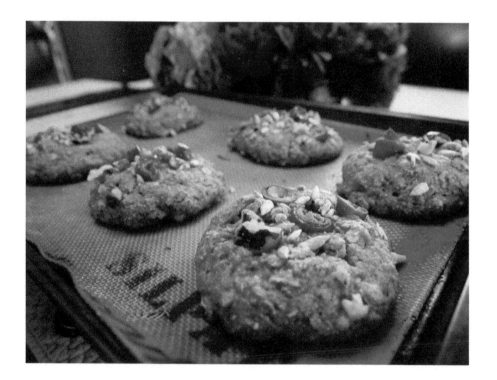

Vegan Breakfast Biscuits

Preparation Time: 10 minutes

Cooking Time: 10 min

Servings: 6

Ingredients:

2 cups Almond Flour

1 tbsp Baking Powder

¼ teaspoon Salt

½ teaspoon Onion Powder

½ cup Coconut Milk

¼ cup Nutritional Yeast 2 tbsp Ground Flax Seeds

¼ cup Olive Oil

Directions:

1.   Preheat oven to 450F.

2.   Whisk together all ingredients in a bowl.

3.   Divide the batter into a pre-greased muffin tin.

4.   Bake for 10 minutes.

Nutrition: calories 432 fat 5 carbs 13 protein 8

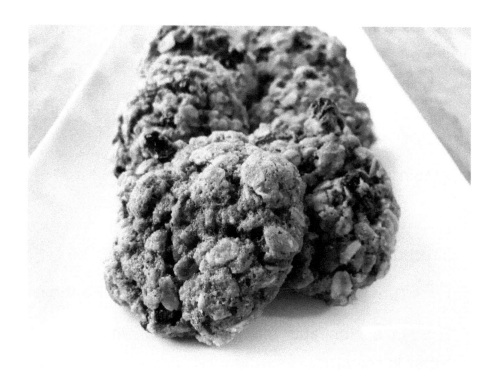

Orange French Toast

Preparation Time: 5 minutes

Cooking Time: 30 minutes

Servings: 8 servings

Ingredients:

2 cups of plant milk (unflavored) Four tablespoon maple syrup 11/2 tablespoon cinnamon

Salt (optional)

1 cup flour (almond)

1 tablespoon orange zest 8 bread slices

Directions:

1.   Turn the oven and heat to 400 degrees F afterward.

2.   In a cup, add Ingredients: and whisk until the batter is smooth.

3.   Dip each piece of bread into the paste and permit to soak for a couple of seconds.

4.   Put in the pan, and cook until lightly browned.

5.   Put the toast on the cookie sheet and bake for ten to fifteen minutes in the oven until it is crispy.

Nutrition: Calories: 129 Fat: 1.1g Carbohydrates: 21.5g Protein: 7.9g

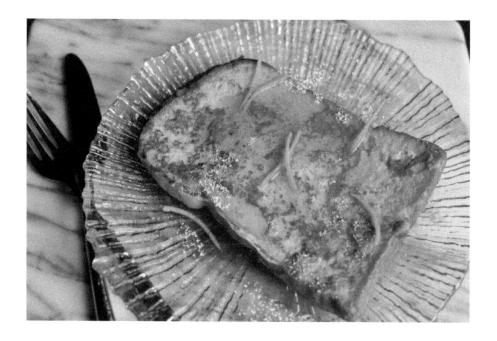

Chickpea Omelet

Preparation Time: 10 minutes

Cooking Time: 30 minutes

Servings: 3 servings

Ingredients:

2 cup flour (chickpea)

11/2 tsp onion powder 11/2 tsp garlic powder

1/4 teaspoon pepper (white and black) 1/3 cup yeast

1 tsp baking powder 3 green onions (chopped)

Directions:

1.   In a cup, add the chickpea flour and spices.

2.   Apply 1 cup of sugar, then stir.

3.   Power medium-heat and put the frying pan.

4.   On each omelet, add onions and mushrooms in the batter while it heats.

5.   Serve your delicious Chickpea Omelet.

Nutrition: Calories: 399 Fat: 11.1g Carbohydrates: 11.5g Protein: 7.9g

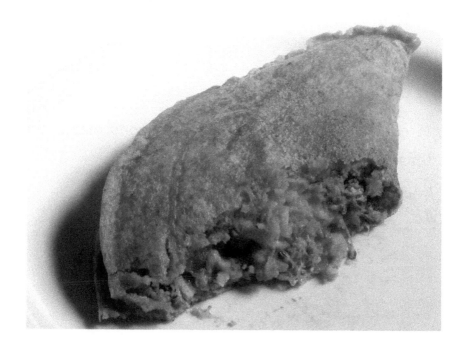

Banana Oatmeal Protein Pancakes

Preparation time: 5 minutes

Cooking time: 15 minutes

Servings: 2

Ingredients:

1½ cups unsweetened plant-based milk 1 cup quick oats

1 banana

½ cup vital wheat gluten

½ cup whole wheat flour 2 tablespoons maple syrup 2 teaspoons vanilla extract

1 teaspoon pink Himalayan salt

Optional Toppings:

Sliced bananas Pecans

Hulled hemp seeds

Maple syrup

Directions:

1. Pu together all the ingredients in a food processor, except the optional toppings and mix until smooth.

2. Use a ¼-cup measuring cup to pour ⅙ of the batter into a non-stick skillet over medium heat. Turn when the edges are browning. Repeat with the remaining batter.

3. Serve immediately with your favorite toppings (if using) or store the pancakes in the refrigerator for up to 3 days.

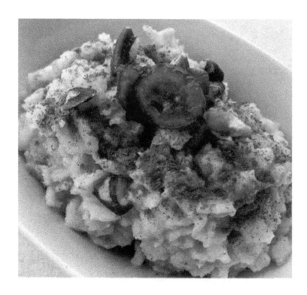

Breakfast French Toast

Cook time: 6 minutes

Servings: 1

Ingredients:

slices bread, gluten-free 2 teaspoons cinnamon

2 tablespoons flaxseed, ground 6 oz. soy milk

2 teaspoons vanilla extract

scoop vegan protein powder

Directions:

1. Mix cinnamon, flaxseed, soy milk, vanilla extract, and protein powder in a deep baking dish. Deep the bread slices into the mixture to coat.
2. Preheat a non-stick frying pan over medium heat and toast the bread for 3 minutes per side. Enjoy!

Dairy-Free Pumpkin Pancakes

Cooking time: 10 minutes

Servings: 12

Ingredients:

1-cup all-purpose flour

1   teaspoons baking powder
½ cup pumpkin puree 1 egg

1   tablespoons chia seeds
3 tbsp coconut oil, melted, slightly cooled 1 cup almond milk

2 teaspoons vanilla extract 1 tablespoon white vinegar
1 tablespoon maple syrup

1 teaspoon pumpkin pie spice

½ teaspoon kosher salt

Instructions:

2. In a bowl, put together vinegar and almond milk. Let rest for 5 minutes.

3. Mix flour, baking powder, baking soda, chia seeds, pumpkin pie spice, and salt in a separate bowl.

4. Whisk eggs into the almond milk, then stir in pumpkin puree, coconut oil, vanilla, and maple syrup.

5. Put together the wet ingredients with the dry ones and mix until blended. Add in more almond milk if the batter is thick.

6. On a medium-heat, place a non-stick frying pan. Scoop out 1/3 of the batter and pour it into the pan. Cook for 1 minute, then flip to the other side and cook until golden brown. Do this with the remaining batter and serve.

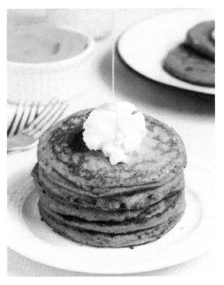

Blueberry Bars

Cook time: 5 minutes

Servings: 16

Ingredients:

½ cup dried blueberries 1 ½ cups rolled oats

¾ cup whole almonds 1/3 cup ground flaxseed 1/3 cup walnuts

¼ cup sunflower seeds

½ cup pistachios 1/3 cup pepitas

¼ cup apple sauce 1/3 cup maple syrup 1 cup almond butter

Instructions:

1. In a bowl, mix rolled oats, blueberries, almonds, flaxseed, walnuts, sunflower seeds, pistachios, and pepitas.

2. Stir in apple sauce and maple syrup. Mix in almond butter, then pour the batter into a baking sheet

lined with parchment paper. Firmly press down the batter using your palms, then spread evenly.

3.   Refrigerate for 1 hour. Remove from the freezer afterward and lift the battery from the pan by lifting from the paper. Place on a working surface and gently remove the paper. Cut the dough into 16 bars and serve.

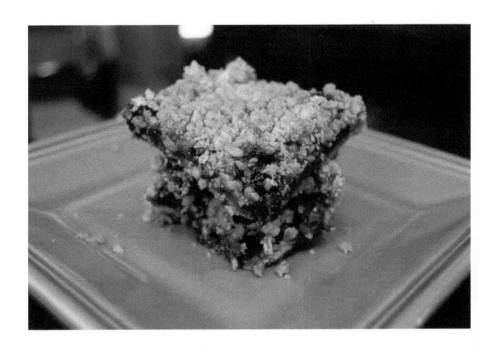

Breakfast Quinoa with Apple Compote

Prep time: 10 minutes

Cook time: 35 minutes

Serves 4

Quinoa:

1½ cups quinoa, rinsed and drained 1 cinnamon stick

Salt, to taste

Apple Compote:

½ cup date molasses

1 cup dates, pitted and chopped

4 apples, peeled, cored, and diced 1 teaspoon ground cinnamon

Pinch ground nutmeg

Zest and juice of 1 lemon

Make the Quinoa

1. Bring to boil 3 cups of water over high heat. Add the quinoa, cinnamon stick, and salt. Cover the pot,

bring the mixture back to a boil, reduce the heat to medium, and cook the quinoa is tender. Remove the cinnamon stick before serving.

Make the Apple Compote

2. Place the date molasses in a small saucepan and bring it to a boil over medium heat. Add the dates, apples, cinnamon, nutmeg, lemon zest, and juice, cook for 15 minutes.

3. To serve, divide the quinoa among 4 individual bowls and top with the apple compote.